Health Is Wealth for Women

Anti Inflammatory Diet, Fibroids, Thyroids, Birth Control, Cancer and Healthy Lifestyle

Rachel Hall

Table of Contents

Introduction

Congratulations on purchasing *Health Is Wealth for Women,* and thank you for doing so.

The following chapters will discuss the conditions plaguing women's health, how medical professionals generally treat these conditions, the role that day-to-day activities play in these health concerns, and how to use this knowledge to prevent and treat these conditions at home.

What makes this information so important is that women don't always know what lies ahead. Women have often been prescribed hormonal birth control to treat various conditions and symptoms related to those conditions, such as Endometriosis and Fibroids, aside from just preventing pregnancy. However, the risk of cancer and other disorders increases with the use of hormone-altering contraception.

Healthcare professionals are doing what they can, but there are ways that you can take your health into your own hands. Knowledge is the most important weapon. This book is here to arm you with the knowledge you need to take control of your health, understand the risk factors, and help you learn holistic measures to prevent and treat conditions, limiting extreme healthcare treatments, such as surgery.

This is a journey through these conditions, the risk factors, the treatments, and, most importantly, what you can do to help yourself. There are plenty of books discussing this subject on the market, thanks again for choosing this one! Every effort was made to ensure it is full of as much useful and digestible information as possible. Please enjoy!

Chapter 1: Fibroids Uncovered

Tumors Affecting Women

Just a quick overview to cover all bases and make this less complicated:

Before we dive into these chapters, we need a basic understanding of the reproductive organs because we will refer to them going forward. Please refer to the diagram and definitions below as a reference.

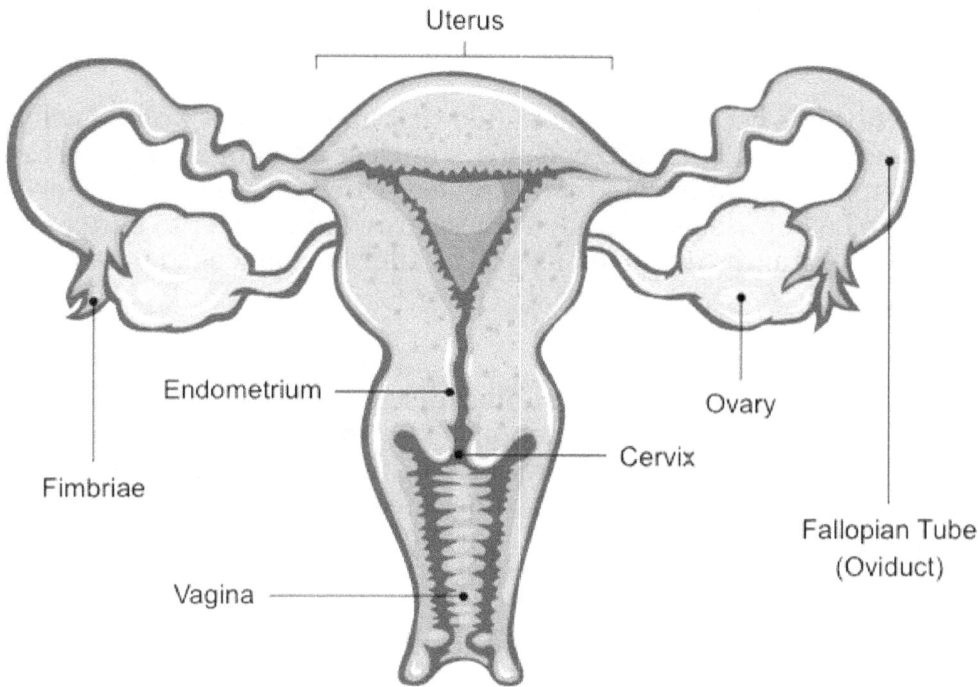

Uterus: The part of the women's reproductive system where a baby is conceived and carried throughout pregnancy (the inside is also known as the womb)

Vagina: The external portion of a women's reproductive system, connected to the cervix, where the penis enters to impregnate a woman

Cervix: The narrow connection from the vagina to the uterus

Fallopian Tube (sometimes referred to as an oviduct): The tube in which the ovum (egg) travels from the ovary to the uterus (a healthy reproductive system has two)

Ovary: The part of the female reproductive system where ova (eggs) are produced (a healthy reproductive system has two)

Endometrium: The lining of the uterus (this is what thickens during the menstrual cycle in order to prepare for possible pregnancy)

Fimbriae: The fringe at the end of the fallopian tube where it connects to the ovary

Now that we've gotten the housekeeping out of the way, let us move on to a greater understanding of Health Is Wealth for Women.

There are many disorders that are specifically affecting women's health. Among them are various cancers, such as Cervical and Uterine Cancer and conditions, such as Endometriosis and Fibroids. Throughout the next few chapters, we will discuss many of these conditions in detail to give you a base overview of each and an understanding of how our day-to-day choices and the push for medical intervention continue to affect women's health.

We start with fibroids because it is estimated that up to 70% of women will develop fibroids in their lifetime. Their direct cause is unclear and not all fibroids cause negative symptoms, so it may go undetected or untreated. However, their prevalence is alarming. Women need to be knowledgeable about these growths in order to better equip themselves to detect and treat them, as well as alter life choices to potentially prevent them or reduce their size.

Fibroids

Perhaps one of the most common and under-discussed conditions affecting women's health is the fibroid. A fibroid is a tumor, also known as an abnormal growth, that can grow in the uterus. They can cause heavy menstruation and moderate-severe pain depending on how large they grow, but sometimes cause no changes at all. This means that some women may have fibroids and not even know. In most instances, fibroids are benign, which means they are not cancerous.

It is important to know the names used by healthcare professionals when discussing fibroids, so you know that they are talking about the same thing. Fibroids can be known as leiomyomas, myomas, uterine myomas, and/or fibromas. These names are synonymous with fibroids, but there are four distinct types of fibroids to be familiar with. The distinguishing characteristics to determine the difference between each kind of fibroid is where they develop in the uterus.

Types of Fibroids

Intramural fibroids are myomas that grow inside the wall of the uterus. These are the most commonly diagnosed as they can grow large and make their way to the woman's womb.

The second kind is called a Subserosal fibroid. These grow outside of the uterus (also now as the serosa, where the name comes from). If these grow vast enough, they can make it seem as though your womb is disproportionately larger on one side or area.

Thirdly, Subserosal fibroids can change shape and grow what looks like the stem of a flower at the base of the myoma. These are called Pedunculated fibroids.

The last is known as a Submucosal fibroid. The middle part of the uterus is known as the myometrium. This is where Submucosal fibroids grow. These are the least common.

Each of these fibroids is pictured below to give you a better idea of what was discussed above.

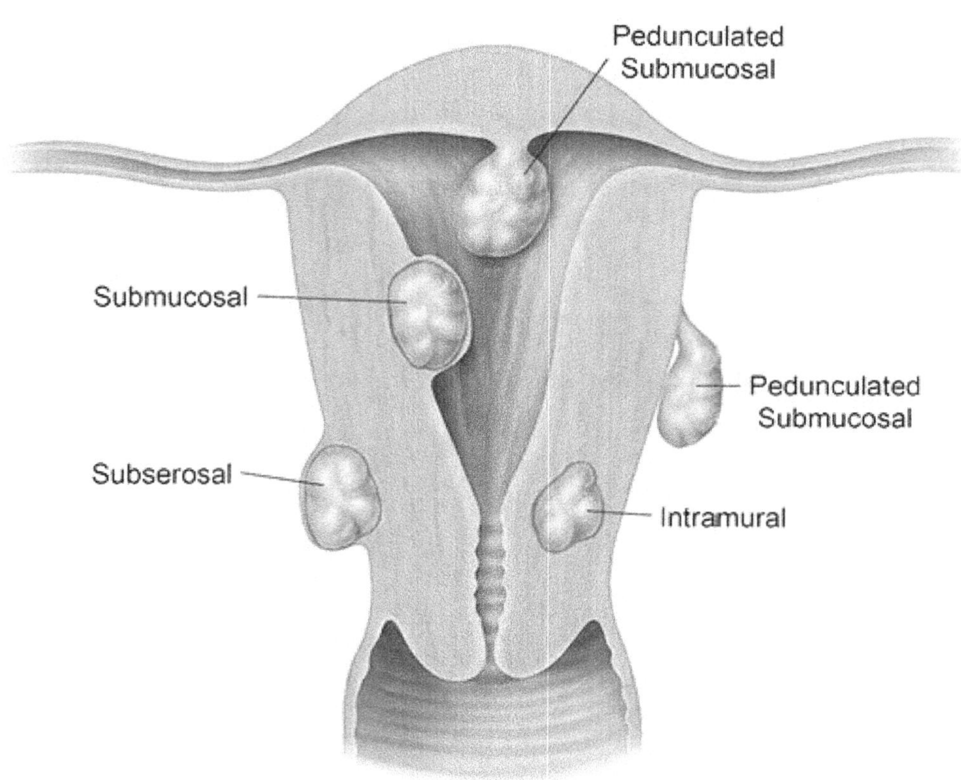

Risk Factors and Symptoms

Many factors contribute to the development of fibroids, including family history, hormones, and pregnancy. While it may be the case that estrogen and progesterone kickstart the growth of these tumors (which is why they may grow faster in pregnancy), there is no clear cause as to why this is the case.

Symptoms of fibroids vary, but may include: heavy menstruation and/or worsened cramping, longer menstrual cycles, pain in the pelvis, lower back discomfort and/or pain, increased urgency or frequency of urination, discomfort and/or pain during intercourse, pressure or swelling in the lower abdomen, and difficulty during pregnancy, labor, and/or delivery.

Those considered to have a greater risk of growing fibroids women that are age 30 or over, pregnant women, those with a family history of myomas, and African Americans. Obesity has been linked to the development of fibroids as well, and this will be discussed more in future chapters.

Chapter 2: Surgical and Non-Surgical Treatment of Fibroids

How Fibroids Are Treated By Medical Professionals

Now that we have a base understanding of what fibroids are, how they affect women, and the different kinds, let's review the treatments used by medical professionals to treat fibroids. There are three ways these treatments can be broken down: watchful waiting, surgical procedures, and drug therapy. Watchful waiting is the delay of treatment coupled with frequent pelvic exams and ultrasounds to monitor the growth of fibroids. If watchful waiting proves that there is more that needs to be done, surgical and/or drug therapy will be recommended. These possible treatments are reviewed below.

Hysterectomy

Hysterectomy is a surgical procedure in which the uterus is removed completely from the woman. This is generally chosen for women that experience heavy bleeding, sometimes requiring transfusions or causing severe anemia and are close to entering menopause, or for women that are already post-menopausal. Medical professionals may recommend a hysterectomy if other, less-invasive measures have not helped. However, a hysterectomy is a common recommendation for any woman with a condition affecting her uterus if she is passed the child-bearing years.

There are two different types of hysterectomies. The first is a total hysterectomy, which is the taking out both the uterus with the cervix at once. The second is known as a subtotal hysterectomy or supracervical hysterectomy, which is when the uterus is taken out while the cervix remains.

A little history on the word hysterectomy: It is believed that the uterus (and the rest of the female reproductive organs) are no longer necessary after child-bearing years even today, though the absence of these organs can have terrible effects on hormonal balance and increase the risk of stroke and other conditions. The word "hysteria" was a diagnosis given to women by psychiatrists and psychologists to cover behaviors peculiar to women. The idea that this "abnormality" in behavior could be reversed or treated by removing the uterus, since this is where the behavior was said to have stemmed from, is how the hysterectomy came about.

Myomectomy

A myomectomy is a grouping of procedures used to remove fibroids. There are three different procedures in this group. The first is a hysteroscopy. This procedure uses a scope inserted into the uterus through the vagina to remove fibroids. The second is a laparotomy, which removes the fibroids through a small incision in the abdomen and sometimes uterus. The last is a laparoscopy. This last procedure uses a laparoscope, a tube equipped with a high-powered light, and a special camera that is inserted through one of two small incisions in the abdomen and a catheter that is inserted through the second incision to remove the fibroids.

Oophorectomy

An oophorectomy is a surgical procedure to remove one or both of the ovaries. It is considered a hysterectomy, though it does not remove the uterus. This is not a typical procedure done for those with fibroids, but it needs to be mentioned as some believe that performing an oophorectomy as a preventative measure for Ovarian Cancer while doing a hysterectomy is beneficial and, therefore, it is worth noting.

There are two distinguishing bilateral (both) oophorectomies. The first is simply a bilateral oophorectomy, which is removing both ovaries. There is also a bilateral salpingo-oophorectomy, which is removing both the ovaries and both fallopian tubes. Either of these techniques can be done in conjunction with the removal of the uterus (hysterectomy).

Uterine Fibroid Embolization

A Uterine Fibroid Embolization (UFE) is much less intrusive and is done via accessing the femoral artery (leg) or the radial artery (wrist) using a catheter introduced through a small incision. Contrast (a dye) is dispensed to show up in an x-ray. This is used to locate the blood supply for the fibroids so it can be blocked, thus preventing the fibroids from growing. Uterine Fibroid Embolization is appropriate for most fibroids except those that are deemed too large.

Endometrial Ablation

Endometrial Ablation is used for small fibroids within the uterus by terminating the lining of the uterus (endometrium). This can be done using heat from radiofrequency, heated fluid, or microwaves. This is less invasive, but women that choose to use this procedure will be risking their ability to get pregnant and carry to term, and increase the risks of complications. Endometrial Ablation may pose a challenge to diagnosing uterine cancer should it develop later on.

Magnetic Resonance Guided Focused Ultrasound

Magnetic Resonance Guided Focused Ultrasound (MRgFUS) is another non-intrusive method like the Endometrial Ablation using heat, but instead of destroying the endometrium, the heat is focused on destroying the uterine fibroids themselves. MRgFUS is recommended for women that have already had children and don't want to have any more or don't plan to do so at all. MRgFUS is also limited to fibroids within the uterus only.

Ultrasound Guided Radiofrequency Ablation

Ablation is the term used for the heat being applied in the two above procedures, and it is used in an Ultrasound Guided Radiofrequency Ablation as well. This time, the heat is applied to the fibroids using the laparoscopic procedure we discussed with the types of myomectomies. Ultrasound is used to find each of the fibroids, and then the radiofrequency device applies the heat to destroy them. This technique can be completed outpatient and is considered low risk.

GnRH Agonists

GnRH Agonists (also known as Gonadotropin-Releasing Hormone Agonists) are a type of hormonal drug therapy used to treat fibroids. They can be dispensed in an implant, monthly injection, or even a nasal spray. GnRH Agonists keep certain reproductive hormones from emitting: luteinizing hormone (LH) and follicle-stimulating hormone (FSH). This prevents ovulation and, therefore, stops the production of estrogen. These are known to reduce fibroids.

Hormonal Contraception

Contraception used in Women's Health for more than just pregnancy prevention is something that is incredibly common. Oral contraceptions do not prevent the growth or prominence of fibroids, but are used to counteract symptoms, such as heavy menstrual bleeding. IUDs (or intrauterine devices) release progestin, which also reduces the bleeding. We will discuss the role of hormonal contraception on Women's Health more in-depth in Chapter 4.

Natural Remedies

Some home remedies have had some success in reducing symptoms of fibroids as well. Examples are acupuncture, yoga, massage, and applying heat to soothe pain. Managing stress and changes in diet have also shown to manage symptoms of fibroids. More details on this will be reviewed in the coming chapters.

Chapter 3: Endometriosis and Thyroids

What Is Endometriosis Exactly, and How Does the Thyroid Tie Into It All?

Before examining some more details on hormonal contraception, natural remedies, and the effects of diet, it is important to understand Endometriosis and conditions that affect the thyroids, as these have effects on hormones and are consequently treated with manipulation of hormones.

Endometriosis

Endometriosis is most easily explained as a condition in which the tissue that usually lines the uterus (which we learned to be named endometrium) sprouts externally from the uterus. The abnormal tissue can grow on the ovaries, fallopian tubes, and/or intestines. The most usual indications include irregular menstruation and pain. Endometriosis is most commonly treated with hormone therapies, including the use of hormonal contraception, to keep symptoms under control. Unfortunately, Endometriosis is a chronic condition. Similar surgical and non-surgical procedures to combat fibroids (as reviewed in Chapter 2) are used to help with this condition as well. Even more unfortunate, Endometriosis is a common diagnosis, with more than 200,000 new cases diagnosed per year in the US alone.

The Thyroid and Women's Health

The thyroid is a small gland that is part of the endocrine system of the body. It is shaped like a butterfly and lies at the base of the neck. The thyroid is particularly in charge of creating hormones and regulating metabolism. Many women experience difficulty with weight fluctuation and hormone regulation, which, oftentimes, can be attributed to disorders of the thyroid.

There are a few disorders that are most common: Hyperthyroidism, Hypothyroidism, Hashimoto's Disease, and Graves' Disease. Hyperthyroidism is plainly an overactive thyroid. Hypothyroidism is an underactive thyroid. Overactive produces and releases too much hormone and underactive produces and releases too little. Hyperthyroidism is most commonly caused by Graves' Disease and Hypothyroidism, by Hashimoto's Disease. Both are autoimmune disorders.

Furthermore, the thyroid is accompanied by four parathyroid glands, and these glands are responsible for managing the distribution of calcium in the blood and bones. Similar to the thyroid, Hyperparathyroidism is a condition in which one or more of the parathyroid glands are affected by a tumor that causes them to release too much of their hormone. This results in too much calcium in the blood, which causes complications.

Of course, these conditions do not rule out the chance that either the thyroid and/or the parathyroid can also be afflicted with cancer. Cancer in either of these glands furthers the imbalance of the hormones they are responsible for, but respond well to traditional treatments generally.

In both thyroid conditions and endometriosis, treatments are most often hormone therapy. This means the chemicals naturally occurring in your body, telling it how to breathe, grow, drink, eat, and be balanced are being artificially altered to combat the symptoms. In the coming chapter, we will dive into hormonal contraception and the role it plays in everyday life, combatting these conditions, and the increased risk of cancer related to their use.

Chapter 4: The Role of Hormonal Contraception

How Hormonal Contraception Contributes to Women's Health

The CDC outlines the prevalence of birth control in the US. Currently, 12.6% of women aged 15-49 are on a birth control pill. 10.3% of women between 15-49 are using a longterm removeable contraception such as an intrauterine device (IUD) or contraceptive implant. These statistics are just of women currently using one of these forms of contraception. In their lifetime, nearly 98% of women have used some type of contraception at some part of their lives, and 62% are currently using some form of birth control (but this includes all forms of birth control, such as condoms and spermicide, as well as surgical sterilization). The most popular choices tend to use some form of hormonal manipulation through the use of synthetic hormones to prevent pregnancy.

Hormonal Contraception Methods

There are three popular forms of contraception that usually manipulate hormones in the woman's body in order to prevent pregnancy: the birth control pill, a long-lasting insertable contraception , such as an intrauterine device or a contraceptive implant, and a contraceptive injection. These forms of contraception work, in simplest terms, by using synthetic hormones (progestin and estrogen) to stop ovulation. No ovulation means no egg for the sperm to fertilize, which means no pregnancy.

The birth control pill is a daily pill taken by a woman for each day of her menstrual cycle. It must be taken at the same time every single day for it to be successful in preventing pregnancy. These generally work by manipulating estrogen and progestin (a synthetic form of progesterone) or just progestin. Some packs come in 21-day setups where the woman doesn't take the pill the 7 days of her menstruation (period). Others are a 28-day pack where there is a pill on those same 7 days that doesn't contain any synthetic hormones to allow for menstruation, but keep them to the routine of taking the pill each day at the same time. There are options that allow for the prevention of menstruation altogether or limit it to fewer times a year. This form of contraception, when taken as prescribed, is considered to be over 90% successful, but does not prevent sexually transmitted diseases (STDs).

Many women are gravitating toward Intrauterine Devices (IUDs) and Contraceptive Implants because these forms of birth control do not require them to remember to take a pill each day at the exact same time. They don't have to carry it around and have their lives cater to this pill.

Intrauterine Devices are small devices that are inserted into a woman's uterus to prevent pregnancy. An IUD is broken down into two types, a copper IUD that doesn't use hormone manipulation and hormonal IUDs. There is only one brand of the copper IUD approved by the FDA, and it doesn't use hormones. It can stay implanted to protect from pregnancy for up to 12 years. There are many more choices when it comes to hormonal IUDs, and they range from 3-7 years of protection from pregnancy. These work by manipulating the hormone of progesterone to inhibit the normal movement of the sperm, preventing them from getting to the egg. The hormones can thicken the mucus on the cervix, which will keep sperm from moving on, and can sometimes prevent the ova from leaving the ovary altogether.

IUDs are considered to be more than 99% effective, but this is also attributed to the fact that human error is less likely when a woman does not have to remember to do something at the exact same time each and every day. Like birth control pills, they do not protect against STDs.

Similarly to the IUD, Contraceptive Implants are long lasting. They are small rods inserted into the skin of the upper arm to prevent pregnancy for up to 4 years. Just like the IUD, this form of contraception releases progestin to thicken the mucus of the cervix to inhibit movement of the sperm. It is also considered over 99% effective and does not protect against STDs.

The last form of hormonal contraception we are going to review is the Contraceptive Injection. Much like the birth control pill, it can manipulate either estrogen and progestin or just progestin, but instead of taking a pill daily, the woman needs to get an injection either monthly or every three months. It is just as effective as the others and doesn't protect against STDs.

Manipulating the hormones in the body is not an inconsequential decision. All of these forms of birth control reviewed have side effects, some more serious than others. A popularly positive side effect, though not necessarily safe, of most of these forms of birth control is the lessening of bleeding from or the stopping altogether of menstruation. Other side effects include weight fluctuation, blood clots, headaches, mood swings, spotting between periods, to name a few. There are others, and it varies from the type of contraception. For instance, implanting an IUD requires manual stretching of the cervix that can be painful, and if a woman with an IUD does get pregnant, the risk of ectopic pregnancy (when a pregnancy grows outside of the uterus) increases, which can be fatal to both mother and child.

Estrogen Dominance

Hormones in the body are there to keep each person, male or female, balanced. When levels of one or more hormones are too high or too low, that balance no longer exists, and changes can happen in the body. Specifically, estrogen is responsible for regulating the female reproductive system and developing female characteristics, such as breasts. In men, estrogen is responsible for sex drive (libido) and the maturation of sperm.

When estrogen levels are too low in women, the results could be mood swings, headaches, and weight gain. It can also lead to more serious conditions, such as cardiovascular disease, dementia, and osteoporosis. Even men can have some serious repercussions with too little estrogen, including erectile dysfunction, decreased libido, and possibly an increase in body fat. However, the risk of too much estrogen, or Estrogen Dominance, could have side effects more life-threatening, such as cancer.

Cancer from Estrogen Dominance are known as "estrogenic cancers" and are cancers such as ovarian, uterine, breast, and thyroid. In men, prostate cancer has been linked to Estrogen Dominance as well.

To better understand Estrogen Dominance, we must break down estrogen. Estrogen is actually a group of three hormones that are considered female hormones. These three hormones are estradiol, estriol, and estrone.

Estradiol is the female fountain of youth. It is what keeps women feeling and looking young. Estradiol is accountable for the sex drive and comes from the ovaries in women and testosterone in men. This type of estrogen can ward off cardiovascular disease, osteoporosis, and even cancer.

Estriol is disseminated in the body when a woman is pregnant in order to feed the placenta. There is a link to gut health and a belief that this estrogen also has anti-inflammatory properties. Estriol is not usually found after the woman has delivered her baby.

Estrone is also released from the ovaries like estradiol, but, is responsible for menopause. It changes to the estrone estrogen when it is mixed with testosterone, but it can also be created by fat tissue. It is believed that obesity can put women at risk for some cancers for this reason. It has some positive properties, as estrone can defend the heart and brain, but it also is shown to increase the risk of estrogenic cancers and even has a connection to Type 2 Diabetes.

Hormonal Birth Control and Cancer

We have seen this before in mental health. Individuals taking medications to combat depression that have serotonin or dopamine release responsibilities have shown to be disruptive to the body when the individual ceases taking the medication. This is because the body is no longer responsible for these neurotransmitters, so when the individual comes off the medication, the body does not release them. This can cause the person to have worse symptoms than before the use of the medication.

Similarly, the imbalance of even just estrogen can have some really life-threatening results on the body. Estrogen Dominance is especially detrimental to health as it has been linked to many of the cancers that plague women. When the hormones are synthetically manipulated through the use of hormonal contraception, women are opening more doors for these imbalances because the body no longer knows what the proper amount of estrogen is to secrete and when. This confusion can cause the body to over or under produce estrogen to compensate once the hormones are no longer being altered by the contraception.

Let's follow-up with a quick review of what cancers affect women, in particular, to gain a greater understanding of them as we continue on to discuss how to naturally help our bodies.

Breast Cancer

Breast cancer is a well-known condition afflicting women's health (and some men as well). Cancer occurs when old cells that should die do not. Instead, these old cells grow and create abnormal new tissues known as tumors. In the case of breast cancer, these malignant cells and tumors grow in the breast or surrounding tissue.

There are five forms of breast cancer outlined by the National Breast Cancer Foundation, Inc.Ductal Carcinoma In Situ (DCIS) is cancer found in the milk ducts and is considered non-invasive. Contrastly, Invasive Ductal Carcinoma (IDC) is breast cancer that started in the milk ducts and spread. Metastatic Breast Cancer (MBC and AKA Stage 4 Breast Cancer) is detected when cancer has already spread to somewhere else in the body. Inflammatory Breast Cancer (IBC) is known for being aggressive and can spread to the skin and lymph vessels in the breast. Triple Negative Breast Cancer (TNBC) is explained as cancer cells testing negative for the hormones estrogen, progesterone, and HER-2.

Symptoms of breast cancer include breast discomfort or pain, inverted nipples, lumps in the breast, nipple discharge, and/or redness/swelling of the lymph nodes. Treatments are chemotherapy, radiation, and surgery most often.

That was quite a bit of information, but it was necessary. Take note of the similarity between the hormones mentioned in that last breast cancer type and the fibroids we discussed earlier. Estrogen and progesterone levels are key factors in these conditions.

According to medical professionals, early intervention is usually the best way to diagnose and treat breast cancer. It is recommended that all women give themselves regularly, monthly breast exams, and women 55 and older have mammograms every other year (45 and older and annually for those with a higher risk of breast cancer).

Cervical Cancer

Cervical cancer is diagnosed when the cancerous cells form in the cervix. It is believed that strains of Human Papillomavirus (HPV) are usually what cause cervical cancer. This is why women are recommended to have regular exams to check for this virus.

There are two types of cervical cancer: Squamous Cell Carcinoma and Adenocarcinoma. Squamous cells are the cells lining the outer part of the cervix touching the vagina. Squamous Cell Carcinoma occurs when cancer begins in the squamous cells. This is the more common of cervical cancers. Adenocarcinoma starts in the cells lining the cervical canal.

Symptoms of cervical cancer include pain during intercourse, unusual vaginal bleeding, vaginal discharge, pelvic pain, difficulty urinating, swollen legs, kidney failure, pain in the bones, weight loss, loss of appetite, and fatigue. Treatments include chemotherapy, hysterectomy (please refer to Chapter 2 for more details), and targeted therapy.

Ovarian Cancer

Ovarian cancer affects the ovaries. What is so dangerous, especially about ovarian cancer, is that it most often flies under the radar until it has infected far passed the ovaries into the pelvis and belly. The reason for this is that ovarian cancer does not present with symptoms until the later stages. Even in later stages, the symptoms are not generally indicative of ovarian cancer presenting as loss of appetite and a decrease in weight. The good news is that this is a rarer cancer and generally affects fewer than 200,000 US women per year.

The primary symptoms of ovarian cancer are abdominal swelling, weight loss, pain or discomfort in the pelvis, change in bowel movements, becoming full faster than usual, and increased frequency to urinate.

There are three types of ovarian cancer: epithelial tumors, stromal tumors, and germ cell tumors. Epithelial tumors are the most commonly diagnosed version of ovarian cancer, and it starts in the thin layer of tissue on the outside of the ovaries. Stromal tumors begin in the tissue that houses the cells responsible for producing hormones. Germ Cell tumors are the least likely of ovarian cancers. This form begins in the cells responsible for producing the ova.

Oophorectimies with or without hysterectomies (refer to Chapter 2 for more information) are among the most common forms of surgical treatment. However, ovarian cancer can be treated with chemotherapy or targeted therapy, as well.

Uterine Cancer

Uterine cancer is also less common, infecting less than 200,000 women in the US per year, similar to ovarian cancer. It begins in the uterus, usually with the abnormal cancer cells growing in the endometrium. Those most at risk are listed as women that are overweight, have never had children, or start their menstrual cycles younger than average.

The most common symptoms are vaginal bleeding, especially after menopause, vaginal discharge, pain when urinating, pain when having sex, and/or pain. The most common treatment is to do a hysterectomy (please refer to Chapter 2 for more information), but hormone therapy is a less invasive option that involves the use of usual progesterone to kill the uterine cancer cells because the abundance of estrogen is causing the cancer cells to grow.

Now that we have a base understanding of the estrogenic cancers and cancers affecting women, in particular, we can discuss how to help prevent these conditions naturally. In the next chapter, we will revisit each of these cancers as well as some other conditions to look more closely at prevalence, risk factors, and risk groups.

Chapter 5: Statistics

Why We Should Pay Attention

In this chapter, we are going to look at the frequency of the conditions we have reviewed, as well as the who is most at risk and, when able, why. This knowledge helps us understand why we should be attentive to Women's Health and leads us to how we can help heal ourselves.

Fibroids

Fibroids are usually benign tumors found in or on the uterus (discussed in detail in Chapter 1). As mentioned in Chapter 1, it is believed that up to 70% of women have or will have fibroids in their lifetime, but the statistics are a little vague since many women will not have symptoms or their symptoms are mild. According to WomensHealth.Gov, between 20% and 80% will have fibroids by the time they are 50 years of age.

The occurrence of fibroids seems to increase with age and is most prevalent in women in their 30s and 40s. It is common for fibroids to shrink after menopause, most likely due to the change in estrogen, and estrogen is what feeds the fibroids.

Women that have family members that have a history of fibroids are more at risk of developing fibroids themselves. In fact, if a woman's mother has had fibroids in her lifetime, the woman is approximately three times as likely to grow fibroids than another woman that doesn't have anyone in her family with the condition. Furthermore, African Amerian women are more at risk for the growth of fibroids than Caucasian women.

Lastly, obesity and eating habits also play a role in the growth of fibroids. Overweight women are more at risk, and obese women may be increasing their risk by two to three times. Additionally, women that eat quite a bit of red meat and/or ham have been noticed to have higher rates of fibroid development, and those that eat many green vegetables seem to have less risk.

Endometriosis

According to WomensHealth.org, it is believed that 11% of women in the US between the ages of 15 and 44 have endometriosis and are believed to be most usual for women in their 30s and 40s. Endometriosis can make it difficult for women to get pregnant, but symptoms are known to subside once a woman with endometriosis does get pregnant.

Hispanic women and African American women are about 50% less likely to have endometriosis rather than Caucasian women. Asian women are more than 50% more likely to be diagnosed with endometriosis.

While the cause of endometriosis is unknown, there are a few risk factors that are believed to be associated. The most likely risk factor for endometriosis is called retrograde menstrual flow. This is when the tissue discharged during menstruation backflows through the fallopian tube or tubes into other areas of the body, mainly the pelvis.

Some other likely risk factors include family history of the endometriosis, history of surgery in the abdomen (such as a cesarean section or hysterectomy), immune system disorders, and hormones. There is a trend we have already touched on about the hormone estrogen being responsible for many of the conditions plaguing women. Endometriosis is no different, and the link between estrogen and endometriosis is there.

Exercise, avoiding alcohol, avoiding caffeine, and maintaining a healthy body weight are recommendations made by medical professionals to prevent or naturally help the diagnosis of endometriosis. Also, talking to your healthcare professionals about birth control methods and reducing the intake of synthetic estrogen may help prevent and/or treat endometriosis.

Thyroid Conditions

As discussed in Chapter 3, conditions afflicting the thyroid, and the parathyroid can disrupt the balance in the body. Women are generally more commonly diagnosed with thyroid conditions rather than men, which is why they are especially included in this discussion (about one in every eight women). In fact, the risk of thyroid conditions increases right after pregnancy or menopause, two milestones in a women's life that require the flooding and ebbing of hormones, especially estrogen.

According to the American Thyroid Association, more than 12% of Americans will acquire a thyroid condition (that's about 20 million people in America alone believed to have a thyroid condition), and perhaps up to 60% of those people don't even know they are afflicted.

Undiagnosed or poorly treated thyroid conditions could put those afflicted at a higher risk for conditions such as cardiovascular disease, osteoporosis, and even infertility. Pregnant women under the same conditions are additionally more at risk for miscarriage, preterm delivery, and/or giving birth to a child having severe developmental conditions.

Race seems to play a hand in the development of the autoimmune conditions Graves; Disease and Hashimoto's Disease. It appears that African Americans and Asians are much more likely to develop Graves' Disease, while Caucasians have much more risk of contracting Hashimoto's Disease, according to a study don from 1997-2011.

While obesity and weight are not usually associated with causing thyroid conditions, the thyroid is responsible for weight consistency and regulating the metabolism, so many of those plagued with a thyroid disorder experience weight fluctuation, especially weight gain.

Breast Cancer

According to the Center for Disease Control and Prevention (CDC), amid American women, breast cancer is the second most diagnosed form of cancer, making it one of the most terrifying threats facing Women's Health. With 124.2 women total for every 100,000 contracting breast cancer, it's no wonder that is. The statistics for African American and Caucasian women occurrences are virtually the same, but the risk does go down a little bit for those that are Asian or Hispanic.

The risks are vast, such as aging, reproductive history, and genetic mutations, as well as obesity and the use of hormones. Some of these risk factors are not something that a woman can change, but there are a few that she can. Let's break them down.

Age is a risk factor; the statistics showing that most breast cancer is diagnosed after age 50. Those that have inherited the BRCA1 and BRAC2 genes are more at risk for developing not only breast cancer, but ovarian cancer too. Similarly, family history of breast cancer also increases the risk of contracting, increasing risk based on the degree the relative that has had breast cancer is from the woman (first-degree is a mother, sister, daughter, for example).

Furthermore, personal history of breast cancer or other breast conditions also increases the risk of breast cancer. So for instance, if you had cancer in one breast, you are more at risk of contracting it again in that breast or the other. Even the radiation used to treat the first bout of breast cancer can increase the risk of contracting breast cancer again.

Reproductive history plays a role because those that started menstruation before age 12 and/or started menopause after age 55 increase the time they have been exposed to certain hormones (like estradiol estrogen discussed in Chapter 4). These hormones are partially responsible for breast cancer.

Dense breasts are considered breasts that have more connective tissues than fatty tissues in the breast. The connective tissue is more difficult to see tumors through when doing a mammogram, making dense breasts not only a greater risk for breast cancer but also a problem for early detection, which is incredibly vital in helping those afflicted survive and recover.

Lastly, there is an increased risk noted for those that have been given the drug diethylstilbestrol (DES) while pregnant or born to a pregnant woman that has taken this drug in the US between the years 1940 and 1971. The drug was dispensed to prevent miscarriage.

Contrastly, there are risk factors that you have more power to change than the risks previously mentioned. These risk factors have more to do with lifestyle choices. Women that are more physically active are less likely to get breast cancer. Women that are overweight or obese, especially after menopause, are more likely to get breast cancer. Additionally, drinking alcohol increases the risk of breast cancer with more alcohol that is regularly consumed.

The choices a woman makes regarding reproduction, and the term of her pregnancies also affect the risk of having breast cancer. Women that had their first pregnancy after the age of 30 are more at risk. Woman that breastfed their baby(ies) are less at risk. Never carrying a pregnancy to term is also considered a risk factor.

Lastly, taking hormones in some form or another raises the possibility of breast cancer. This includes women that take part in hormone replacement therapy during menopause is one way. Some birth control pills have also shown to increase the risk, especially if they are taken for five or more years. Both of these require the use of synthetic hormones, mainly estrogen and progesterone, to manipulate the body, and, as reviewed in Chapter 4, this can cause the body to be unable to regulate hormones for itself and increase the risk of estrogenic cancers.

Cervical Cancer

Cervical cancer is more rare than breast cancer. It affects about 7.7 women out of every 100,000 in the US, according to the CDC. African American women are slightly more at risk of contracting cervical cancer than Caucasian women, but Asian women are less likely than either to have cervical cancer. The most at risk, above all, are Hispanic women.

Cervical cancer is almost always contracted from Human Papillomavirus or HPV. This is an STD that is very common. Not all strains of HPV are known to cause cervical cancer, but some are. For most women, it will even go away on its own, but it can last in the system for quite a long time. Those that don't recover on their own are more at risk for cervical cancer.

While cervical cancer is most often associated with HPV, there are a few other factors that can increase the risk of cervical cancer. Those with HIV or AIDs, or another immune-compromising disorder are more at risk for cervical cancer. Those that smoke are more at risk. Those that have many sexual partners and/or have given birth to three or more children are more at risk. Lastly, and like some of the other conditions we have reviewed, using hormone-altering contraception like the birth control pill for five or more years increases the risk of cervical cancer.

Ovarian Cancer

Ovarian cancer is a bit more prevalent than cervical cancer, with 10.3 out of every 100,000 having ovarian cancer in the US as per the CDC. Caucasian and then Hispanic women are more likely than African American and Asian women to get ovarian cancer. However, the CDC does point out that those with an Eastern European or Ashkenazi Jewish background are most at risk for ovarian cancer.

It is necessary to mention that many of the women in jeopardy of contracting ovarian cancer are also in jeopardy of contracting breast cancer. As discussed above, the genetic mutation inherited from the BRCA1, and BRAC2 genes make the carriers more susceptible to breast cancer and ovarian cancer.

Additionally, those more at risk for ovarian cancer include women that are over 50, those with a family history (especially first-degree relatives) of ovarian cancer, a woman that has had either breast, uterine, or colorectal (colon) cancer, those that have endometriosis, and those that have never given birth or have had trouble getting pregnant.

It has also been shown in some studies that women that have taken estrogen (with or without progesterone) for ten or more years have an increased risk for ovarian cancer. The estrogen is likely the synthetic estrogen found in hormonal contraception, as we have seen.

Uterine Cancer

Uterine cancer is more common than cervical cancer and ovarian cancer, but not as prevalent as breast cancer. According to the CDC, 27.3 out of every 100,000 US women get uterine cancer. It seems to affect African American and Caucasian women in about the same frequency, with Hispanic women being diagnosed slightly less often. Asian women have less cases.

Women at a higher risk of uterine cancer include those that are 50 or older, those that are obese, those that have had trouble getting pregnant, those that have fewer than five periods in a year before menopause, and those having a familial occurrence of uterine cancer, colon cancer, or ovarian cancer in their family history. Furthermore, women that have taken a drug called tamoxifen (used to treat some forms of breast cancer) are at higher risk of uterine cancer, as well. Lastly, women that take estrogen without progesterone for hormone replacement during menopause have higher rates of uterine cancer.

As we have seen, going through these conditions plaguing women, in particular, hormone manipulation, is considered a risk factor more often than not. Most often, that hormone manipulation is from the voluntary and non-medically necessary use of hormonal contraception, as we discussed in Chapter 4. As we move forward, we are going to discuss a few other conditions that are important to review when discussing women's health.

Obesity

Obesity has been mentioned as a risk factor in almost all of the previously discussed conditions. Thyroid conditions were the exception, but diet and exercise are incredibly important for those with thyroid conditions because the thyroid is in charge of the metabolism and excessive weight fluctuation, especially weight gain is likely with a thyroid condition, which could lead to a subsequent condition, such as one of the conditions listed above as well as cardiovascular issues, diabetes, and cholesterol problems.

Roughly 42.4% of the US population is considered obese, according to the CDC. Obesity is considered to be anyone that has a BMI (body mass index) of 30 or higher, but being overweight and not obese is still a common problem as well.

Obesity affects African Americans the most at 49.6%, Hispanics a little less at 44.8%, and then Caucasians at 42.2%, a little less than the Hispanics, but the numbers are incredibly close. Asians have the least frequency of obesity at 17.4%.

The breakdown of age shows that 40% of young adults are obese. Those considered middle-aged are 44.8% obese. Those older than 60 are 42.8% obese.

Lastly, men and women are afflicted with obesity at similar rates, but women of African American descent have the highest rates of obesity in the US.

Diabetes

Diabetes is a chronic condition in which the body either doesn't create enough insulin or can not utilize the insulin it has created. Insulin is the substance in the body released by the pancreas to assist with blood sugar penetration of the cells in the body in order for it to be utilized for energy. When the body does not create a sufficient amount of insulin or the body does not realize how to utilize the insulin the body is making efficiently, there ends up being an abundance of unused sugar in the blood, and it stays in the bloodstream causing complications. Prolonged issues with diabetes leads to heart disease, vision loss, kidney disease, even loss of extremities.

There is no cure for diabetes. However, managing weight, eating healthy, and exercising can help, especially in warding off the condition. There are medications that can help manage blood sugar and insulin injections that can bring down blood sugar as well.

There are three forms of Diabetes: Type 1 Diabetes, Type 2 Diabetes, and Gestational Diabetes.

Type 1 is known as an autoimmune condition and causes the body to stop creating insulin. This type of diabetes affects only 5-10% of the people that have diabetes. Usually, younger members of the population are diagnosed with Type 1 diabetes and there isn't a know prevention method. Those with Type 1 Diabetes are generally insulin-dependent for life.

Approximately 90-95% of those that have diabetes are diagnosed with Type 2 Diabetes. Type 2 occurs usually in older adults, where, over time, they have no longer been able to keep their blood sugar within a normal range, and the body starts to reject the insulin it creates naturally. This type of diabetes is widely believed to be preventable or delayed with weight management, eating healthy, and keeping active. There is a time when those in jeopardy of developing Type 2 Diabetes may be diagnosed as prediabetic. More than one in three adults are considered prediabetic. This occurs when blood sugar is higher than ordinary, but the body is still processing the insulin it makes. Most often, those with a prediabetic diagnosis are able to turn it around with dieting, exercise, and weight loss.

Gestational Diabetes is diabetes, specifically affecting pregnant women that have no history of Type 1 Diabetes nor Type 2 Diabetes. In fact, those that develop gestational diabetes generally stop having the condition following the delivery of the baby, and not all pregnancies for someone with gestational diabetes will bring about gestational diabetes. However, those that have had gestational diabetes are more in danger of ending up with Type 2 Diabetes later in life.

According to the CDC, about 34.2 million people in the US have diabetes (that's about 10.5% of the population). About 88 million adults have prediabetes in the US (that's 34.5 % of the population).

According to the 2020 Diabetes Report done by the CDC, diabetes affects more men than women. Caucasians had the most diagnosed cases in the US in 2018. African Americans and Hispanics have about the same amount of diagnosed cases in 2018, but are significantly less than diagnoses of Caucasians. Asians have the least diagnoses in 2018.

We include the information on diabetes because diabetes is a risk factor for some of the previous conditions reviewed, especially obesity. Obesity poses a risk to almost all of the conditions discussed, and Type 2 Diabetes has been known to be caused specifically by obesity and a sedentary lifestyle.

Cardiovascular Disease

Cardiovascular Disease refers to the group of conditions stemming from the heart. Heart disease, according to the CDC, affects one in every four Americans. The most common form of cardiovascular disease is coronary artery disease, which has the potential to lead to a heart attack.

High cholesterol, high blood pressure, and smoking are the most likely risk concerns. Family history and age are key factors as well.

The most common threat to developing cardiovascular disease is high blood pressure. Your blood pressure is considered high when the blood in the arteries and other blood vessels is too high. High blood pressure is generally able to be reversed by lifestyle changes, but sometimes medication is prescribed. It doesn't pose any symptoms on its own, but can cause not only heart disease, but can pose a threat to the other major organs in the body.

Cholesterol is the thick, waxy material created by the liver or found in foods that can accumulate in the artery walls when excess is consumed. When cholesterol builds up, it narrows the arteries, decreasing the blood flow to the major organs, including the heart and brain.

There are two types of blood cholesterol, and they are Low-Density Lipoprotein (LDL) and High-Density Lipoprotein (HDL). LDL is considered the "bad" cholesterol and HDL, the "good" cholesterol. LDL causes the plaque collection in the arteries that leads to heart disease and other conditions, while HDL cholesterol can actually protect against cardiovascular disease.

Like high blood pressure, high cholesterol does not have any symptoms on its own, but can lead to life-threatening conditions. Both blood pressure and cholesterol should be checked regularly in order to be monitored and maintained, especially in older members of the population.

Diabetes and obesity, as we discussed above, can both also lead to cardiovascular disease. As we learned when discussed diabetes, lifestyle changes can prevent diabetes and reverse prediabetes. Similarly, cardiovascular health can be greatly affected, and heart disease can reverse with management of diet and weight and making sure you get enough exercise. Alcohol use and tobacco use are also risk factors for cardiovascular disease.

Yes, genetics can predispose people to cardiovascular disease, like most other conditions. But lifestyle decisions and regular checkups play a tremendous role in preventing or delaying cardiovascular disease.

Cardiovascular disease is so dangerous as it is considered to be the NUMBER ONE condition causing death in both men and women, and it can be brought about at any age. However, the risk goes up the older an individual gets. It is the top reason of death for African Americans and Caucasians, but is second to cancer in Asians and Hispanics.

Chapter 6: The Anti-Inflammatory Diet

Diet and weight management were the two leading factors in almost every condition discussed in the previous chapter that can be managed on our own. Managing weight and keeping to a healthy diet can prevent and/or lower the risk of almost every single one. And thyroid conditions are the only section where obesity and diet are not listed as risk factors, but do become factors in maintaining health after being diagnosed. Therefore, across the board, diet and weight management are two fo the very most important factors in maintaining health and reversing negative health conditions.

The foods an individual chooses to eat can have therapeutic qualities in much the same way that the opposite foods have effects that create greater challenges in health. Here we are going to discuss how an anti-inflammatory diet can be the most beneficial diet for the maintenance of general health in women and the reversal and prevention of many conditions plaguing women.

Inflammatory Diet vs. Anti-Inflammatory Diet

To start, it is important to understand what inflammation is. Inflammation is the body's response to infection, illness, or injury. So when a person consumes foods that are inflammatory, the body is reacting in a way that is not natural and can become chronic. As we discussed with birth control, if the body is being manipulated to respond in a way that is not natural for the cause, it forgets how to respond appropriately. In the case of chronic inflammation, a person can experience redness, pain, heat, and swelling.

Many of the foods that we eat or the ingredients in the food we eat cause inflammation. Contrastly, foods that reduce inflammation allow the body to react in a natural way to infections, illnesses, and injuries. This means that the body is able to send attention to the parts of the body that need to be healed instead of helping you digest food and reduce inflammation caused by the foods chosen.

The Role of an Anti-Inflammatory Diet in Women's Health

Previously, we discussed many different conditions plaguing women's health and learned that proper diet and weight reduction play a tremendous role in risk prevention as well as even reversing symptoms of conditions. An anti-inflammatory diet helps the body heal by allowing the body to direct the energy needed to the parts of the body that need healing. Therefore, if a woman adheres to an anti-inflammatory diet, she will experience more self-healing. Not to mention, that the foods consistent with an anti-inflammatory diet will aide in weight loss and management, which lowers the risk for other conditions and helps heal the body more.

Food Associated With an Anti-Inflammatory Diet

The question becomes now, what foods are consistent with an anti-inflammatory diet. Below is a chart of some of the foods that make up an anti-inflammatory diet food group and some of the foods to especially pay attention too.

Anti-Inflammatory Foods Groups	Especially
Vegetables	Leafy greens, brussel sprouts, cabbage, cauliflower
Fruits	Berries (darker the better), coconut, lemon, grapefruit, pineapple, mango, avocados, olives
Healthy Fats	Olive oil, coconut oil
Nuts and Seeds	Almonds, hempseed
Grains	Wild rice
Herbs and Spices	Ginger, fenugreek, turmeric, cinnamon
Tea	Green Tea
Water	Spring, distilled

Important to Avoid

As with above, it is important to know what foods are associated with inflammation, so that they can be avoided. It is important to allow your body time to detox from the inflammatory foods before you really see a difference in your body. Detox is short for detoxification. Basically, your body is still going to respond with inflammation in unnecessary and uncomfortable ways until your body detoxifies the cells, and it uses up all that's left of the energy coming from the inflammatory foods. It is important to avoid the foods listed as inflammatory, especially during the detoxification process in order to start your body on the right path to the healing properties.

Inflammatory Food Groups	Especially
Meat	Red meat, processed meats
Dairy	Cheese, eggs, other animal products
Soy	
Refined Carbohydrates	White bread, pasta
Sugar (especially high-fructose corn syrup)	Desserts, sugary drinks
Processed Vegetable and Seed Oils	Soybean oil, canola oil
Trans Fats	Anything listed as partially hydrogenated in the ingredients
Alcohol	In excess
Other	Anything soy and antacids

Chapter 7: Managing Stress and Combatting Women's Health Condition

What Is Stress?

Your body works because of energy. When we discussed Diabetes, we discussed that insulin helps get the sugar into the cells of your body in order to give them energy. When you are experiencing too much stress, your body devotes an enormous amount of precious energy to the stress instead of keeping itself healthy.

Stress is simply emotional or mental tension. It can be good or bad. Bad stress is known as distress, and good stress is known as eustress. Life is stressful, no matter how you look at it. It's not about eliminating stress entirely; it's about managing it properly. This way, your body is putting the energy where it needs to be. You are still healing yourself, but also still experiencing life.

Techniques for Managing Stress

Managing Stress is not easy and takes practice. Some people choose to cover up their stress with drugs or alcohol, but, as we discussed earlier, that only exacerbates the problem. The trick is to find a healthy outlet to let go of stress.

Meditation, Mindfulness, and Breathing Techniques have been proven to help manage stress. Quieting the mind and focusing on something other than the tasks at hand has shown to even make people more productive. Meditation is simply quietly thinking to the self. This can be done in a guided way (there is plenty of free resources online and through smartphone applications to help achieve this on your own), or it can be done by simply sitting quietly, focusing on a word, phrase, or the simple sound of your breathing. Mindfulness is being aware. Practicing Mindfulness can be done by just sitting with yourself while you are eating and actually focusing on the tastes, textures, smells, colors, and even the sounds of chewing, instead of eating while driving or playing on your phone. This can be applied to every seemingly mundane activity. It's much like meditation, where the goal is to take the mind off what is not actually at hand currently. Finally, breathing techniques can help, as well. They can be used in conjunction with the other two or separately. Breathing techniques work on focusing the breath on calming a person down and quiet the mind. Deep breathing is commonly known, but there are many different kinds of breathing techniques, such as alternate nostril breathing and counted breathing.

If sitting quietly is too difficult for you, a suggestion is to put those practices to movement. Yoga is a wonderful way to move the body with the breath in order to stay focused and present. Yoga is an exercise that combines what was discussed above with body postures. Yoga is also healing for the body and is being used as an alternative or long-term solution to physical therapy. Some health insurance are even covering yoga because of its therapeutic qualities.

Sometimes the yoga and meditation world is just too quiet and slow paced for some. Applying mindfulness to hobby or craft is also a wonderful way to reduce stress. Merely do what it is you love! Read a book, paint a picture, build some bookshelves. Whatever it is you enjoy or would like to try doing, do that. Working with the hands, in particular, can be a really wonderful way to relax and quiet the mind.

If you are a more extroverted person, another wonderful way to de-stress is to talk to a friend or get together with some friends. Have a family game night or engage in a group activity that is engaging and doesn't require being under the influence to be fun or interesting. Cooking for the self is therapeutic as a hobby, but cooking for others is its own kind of therapy as well.

Exercise and Stress Reduction

Of course, exercising has also been recognized as a wonderful way to de-stress, and it is a great way to get in shape, reduce the risk, and prevent most of the conditions we discussed in previous chapters. Exercise, much like yoga, can apply a mindfulness or mind-clearing effect while the physical exercise takes over and occupies the mind. Vigorous exercise especially has the power to help with fat and weight loss, the buildup of muscle, and the release of neurotransmitters that are responsible for happiness, such as Dopamine.

Remember, exercise does not need to be at a gym. If you would prefer to play a sport and participate in an outdoor activity like running or walking, that is still exercising. Just make sure you are doing whatever exercise you choose that is appropriate for your body and practice safety precautions.

Sleep and Stress Reduction

Sleep is necessary for every person. Lack of the proper amount of sleep is an epidemic in this world, and almost no one gets their full hours in or has the proper quality of sleep. Your body needs rest in order to operate effectively and have the energy places where it needs to go. Your body, when lacking the proper rest, is stressed, and it can cause you to be irritable and moody, as well as lower your immune system, which fights infections and keeps you healthy.

Most people have poor sleep hygiene. In other words, most people don't practice good sleep routines. The best way to ensure better sleep is to start with creating a routine and reducing practices that prevent sleep. For instance, having a bedtime routine and going to sleep at exactly the same time each night, coupled with waking up at the same time each morning, promotes a rhythm for your body and the likeliness that you will get better quality of sleep. It is important to remember that this routine should be applied to the weekends too.

Other activities that hinder sleep are using your bed for activities other than sleep, such as playing on your phone. Also, playing on your phone is terrible for sleep as the blue light keeps you up, aside from the fact that it keeps your mind busy. It's best not to use your phone or watch TV right before bed.

Lastly, another important thing to note is that eating is for energy. Having an appropriate dinner time is important to sleep hygiene. You don't want to eat too early, making you hungry when you are about to go to sleep. However, you also don't want to eat too late, because the energy from the food can inhibit sleep.

Conclusion: Tying it All Together

Thank you for making it through to the end of *Women's Health: What You Didn't Know and What You Need to Know*, let's hope it was informative and able to provide you with all of the tools you need to achieve your goals whatever they may be.

The next step is to pull it all together! You are now armed with a baseline of knowledge to take your health into your own hands and work on healing yourself. You have the power to reduce your risk to the conditions we discussed here in this book. You have the power to take control of your health and HEAL. We learned that the most important risk factors come from manipulating your body's normal response systems through the use of hormonal contraception and the consumption of inflammatory foods. We learned that weight loss and management, as well as physical activity, are key factors in health maintenance, healing, and the prevention of life-threatening conditions. We learned that the management of stress by taking time to practice self-care and do activities that enjoyable, as well as getting better quality sleep, also play a role in allowing the body to maintain and heal itself naturally. I really hope you enjoyed the information presented and are ready to take the next steps to take back your life and your health.